CANCER AND MODERN SCIENCE™

OVARIAN CANCER

Current and Emerging Trends in Detection and Treatment

JERI FREEDMAN

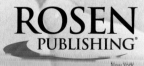

ROSEN
PUBLISHING®
New York

To my niece and nephew, Laura and Matthew Freedman, with love

Published in 2009 by The Rosen Publishing Group, Inc.
29 East 21st Street, New York, NY 10010

Library of Congress Cataloging-in-Publication Data

Freedman, Jeri.
Ovarian cancer: current and emerging trends in detection and treatment / Jeri Freedman.
      p. cm.—(Cancer and modern science)
Includes bibliographical references and index.
ISBN-13: 978-1-4358-5006-4 (library binding)
1. Ovaries—Cancer—Juvenile literature. I. Title.
RC280.O8F74 2009
616.99'465—dc22

                                                                                          2008019943

Manufactured in the United States of America

On the cover: A highly magnified ovarian cancer cell

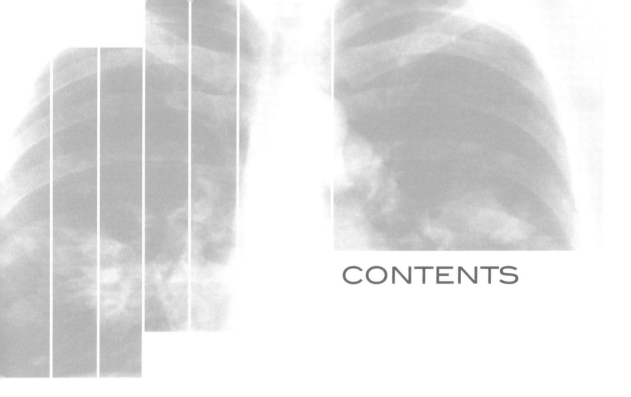

CONTENTS

INTRODUCTION

Ovarian cancer is the second most common form of female reproductive system cancer, after uterine cancer. No one knows the exact cause of ovarian cancer. However, most cases are linked to a defect of one or more genes. Cancer occurs when cells grow out of control. This results in masses of cells called tumors, which can damage surrounding tissue. Ovarian cancer starts in the ovaries, which are the organs that produce a woman's eggs for reproduction. It can also start in the ovaries and spread to other organs.

Ovarian cancer is more common in industrialized nations. It affects about one out of every fifty-five women. Although some cases occur in young women, the majority of cases occur in women between the ages of forty and seventy-nine. It occurs more frequently as women age. Even if it does not affect you directly, it might affect someone in your family.

This book starts with an explanation of ovarian cancer and the genetic defects that cause it. It then looks at how ovarian cancer is diagnosed and treated. Finally, it offers a look at some of the cutting-edge research being done to develop new ways of identifying and treating ovarian cancer.

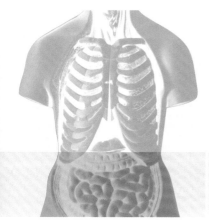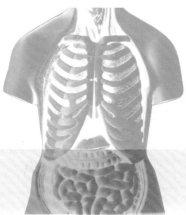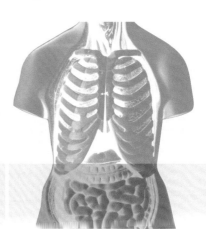

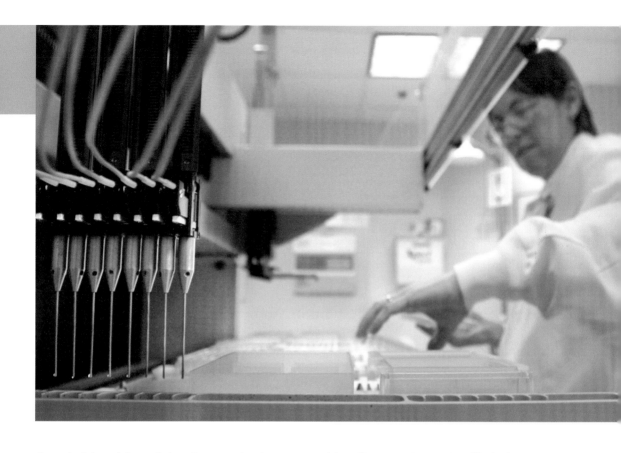

A technician (above) loads samples into a machine for genetic testing. Today's genetic tests can reveal whether a woman is at increased risk for ovarian cancer.

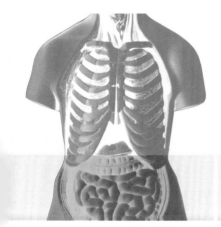
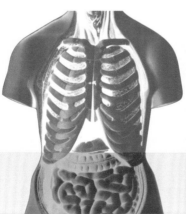
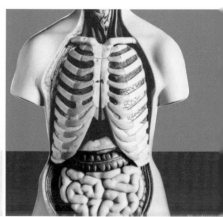

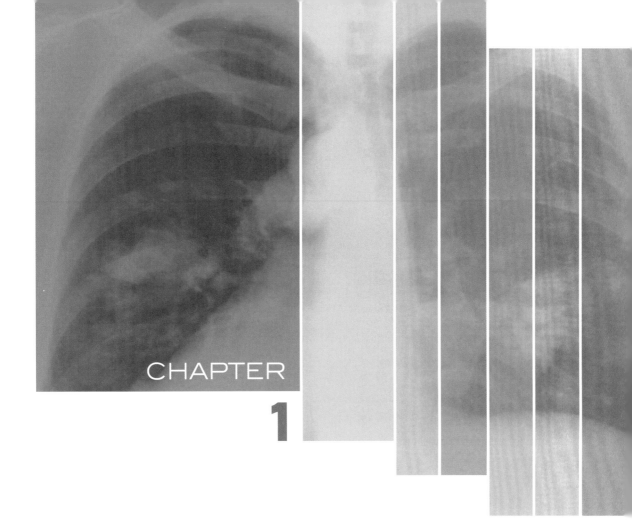

CHAPTER

1

WHAT IS OVARIAN CANCER?

Ovarian cancer is cancer that originates in the ovaries. However, it can spread from the ovaries to other parts of the reproductive system and beyond. In order to understand ovarian cancer, it is first necessary to know something about the female reproductive system.

THE FEMALE REPRODUCTIVE SYSTEM

The internal organs of the female reproductive system include the uterus (womb), ovaries, and fallopian tubes. The ovaries, one on each side of the uterus, are about the size and shape of unshelled almonds.

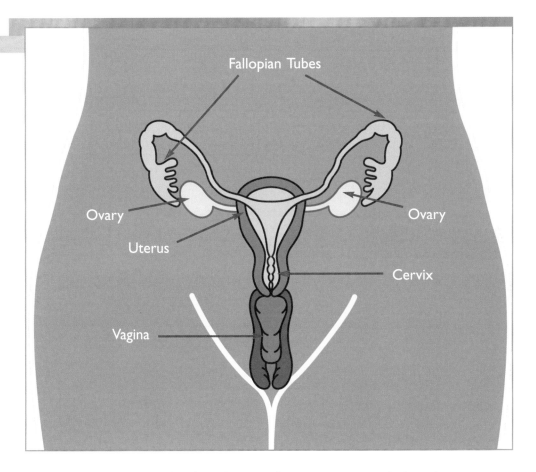

This illustration shows the female reproductive system, including the uterus, ovaries, and fallopian tubes. Eggs travel from the ovaries, through the fallopian tubes, and into the uterus.

They are the organs that produce, store, and release eggs (*ova* is Latin for "eggs"). Men begin producing sperm at puberty and continue to do so throughout their adult lives. Women, on the other hand, are born with all the eggs they will ever have.

Immature egg cells are called oocytes. After puberty, an oocyte matures and is released from an ovary about once a month. The egg travels from the ovary into the fallopian tube and down toward the uterus. If the egg is fertilized by sperm, then it may implant in the uterus and ultimately develop into a fetus. If it is not fertilized, then it will be expelled from the uterus when the woman menstruates (has her period).

An ovary has several layers. The outermost layer of the ovary is made up of epithelial cells. These cells line the inside and outside surfaces of the body and all of its organs. Beneath the ovary's epithelial layer is a layer of connective tissue, or tissue that supports and connects body parts. Beneath that is the major part of the ovary, the cortex. The cortex is filled with follicles, which are round clusters of cells. Each follicle contains one immature egg. A follicle goes through several stages during which it matures and eventually releases the egg. The innermost layer of the ovary is called the medulla. It contains the tissue that attaches the ovary to the abdominal wall and to the blood vessels that bring nourishment to the cells of the ovary and remove waste.

WHAT IS OVARIAN CANCER?

Cancer occurs when cells grow out of control. All the cells in the body function for a period, reproduce, and eventually die. New cells then replace the ones that have died. This life cycle of cells is controlled by genes. Some genes cause cells to grow, and other genes cause them to stop growing and eventually die. When something goes wrong with one of these genes, cells may grow unchecked. This is what happens with cancer.

Cancer cells grow rapidly and live longer than normal cells. They also reproduce, making more cancer cells. Eventually, the cells form a solid mass that grows ever larger. This mass of cells is called a tumor. Tumors can be either benign or malignant. Benign tumors grow slowly and do not spread. Malignant tumors, on the other hand, grow quickly and aggressively spread to other organs.

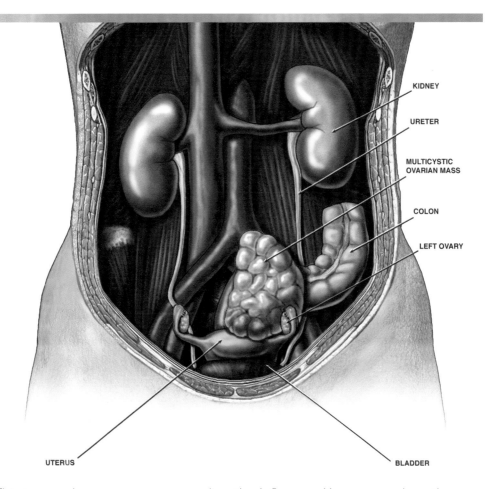

KIDNEY

URETER

MULTICYSTIC OVARIAN MASS

COLON

LEFT OVARY

UTERUS

BLADDER

This image shows a mass surrounding the left ovary. You can see how the growing mass will put pressure on nearby organs, including the uterus. This may eventually affect the functioning of the organs.

When cancer originates in an ovary, it is called ovarian cancer. As the cancerous cells continue to reproduce and grow, they damage the ovarian tissue around them. Cancer can spread from the ovary to other organs of the reproductive system and to other parts of the body as well. The spreading of cancer to other parts of the body is called metastasis.

HISTORY OF CANCER

The earliest recorded cases of cancer come from an Egyptian papyrus dating back to 3000–1500 BCE. The text describes the removal of tumors from the breasts of several patients.

The word "cancer" comes from the Greek word *karkinos*, meaning "crab." The name was coined by Hippocrates (circa 460–370 BCE), the ancient Greek physician who thought the tumors he saw looked like crabs. The ancients did not know what caused cancer. Ancient Egyptians believed it was visited upon people by the gods. Much later, in medieval times, people believed that health was controlled by four substances that circulated in the body: blood, phlegm, yellow bile, and black bile. They called these substances humors. They believed that disease was caused by an imbalance among the four humors. Medieval doctors believed that cancer was caused by too much black bile building up at a place in the body.

In the 1600s, doctors began to develop a more scientific knowledge of the body and its organs. They discovered the lymph nodes, where immune system cells are made, and they learned that lymphatic fluid circulates throughout the body. They started to understand that there was some relationship between the lymphatic system and disease. However, they did not really know about cells, which cannot be seen by the naked eye. They proposed that cancer was caused by lymph fluid collecting and fermenting, or rotting. Several other theories were proposed as causes of cancer, including injury and parasites such as worms.

DISCOVERING CANCER CELLS

Microscopes date back to the 1600s. However, it wasn't until the 1800s that they became powerful enough to allow scientists to use them to study cells. German doctor Rudolph Virchow (1822–1902) observed the difference between normal cells and cancer cells. He also noted the

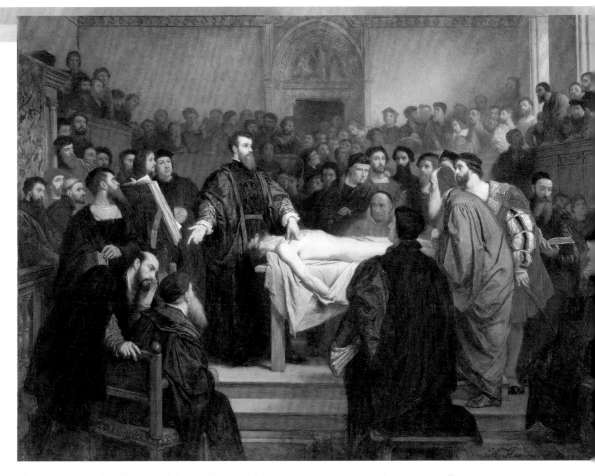

This painting by Edouard Jean Conrad Hamman shows students at a European medical school in the 1500s. By this time, doctors had started to examine dead bodies directly to learn about disease.

changes that take place in cancer cells over time as symptoms of the disease progress. The most common type of ovarian cancer is epithelial cell cancer. In the late 1800s, a German surgeon named Karl Thiersch (1822–1895) first discovered that epithelial cancer was caused by malignant cells spreading throughout the body.

In 1889, an English surgeon named Stephen Paget proposed the "seed and soil" theory of how cancer is spread. He thought that cancer cells could spread through the body from the original site of the cancer but would only take root in organs that had suitable conditions for them to grow. Modern scientists have confirmed Paget's basic theory regarding what happens when cancer cells spread from a tumor to other parts of the body. Their ability to grow in the new location does indeed depend on the conditions of the cells in the new environment.

HISTORY OF CANCER TREATMENT

Surgery improved greatly during the nineteenth century, especially with the development of better anesthesia (pain numbing) and sterilization techniques. During this time, surgical treatment of most cancers involved removing the tumors and the surrounding tissue. In many cases, this radical ("at the root") type of surgery prolonged a patient's life. However, surgery often left the patient deformed and in pain.

Toward the end of the nineteenth century, with increasing knowledge of the way cancer grows and spreads, physicians looked to nonsurgical ways to treat cancer. In 1896, German scientist Wilhelm Conrad Roentgen (1845–1923) invented the X-ray machine. By 1899, X-rays were being used to treat tumors in an early form of radiation therapy.

Chemicals were also used against cancer in a cruder form of modern chemotherapy. The first mention of chemicals being used in this way appears in an 1894 medical textbook by the Canadian physician Sir William Osler (1849–1919). Osler records the use of arsenic to treat cancer.

The development of chemical weapons in World War II (1939–1945) led to major advances in chemotherapy. For example, poisonous mustard gas was used as a weapon because it debilitated and sometimes killed soldiers on the battlefield. While studying the dead bodies of these unfortunate soldiers, doctors discovered that mustard gas actually dissolved

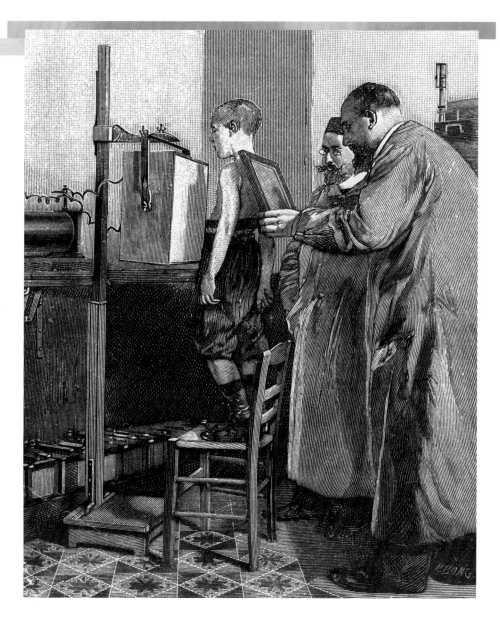

This wood engraving by Richard Bon shows Wilhelm Conrad Roentgen (right) performing an X-ray examination on a boy. Roentgen was awarded the first Nobel Prize in Physics for his work.

lymphatic tissue when inhaled. With this knowledge, researchers Louis S. Goodman and Alfred Gilman pursued the use of mustard gas in treating cancerous tumors. They performed a study using nitrogen mustard, a chemical derived from mustard gas, with very promising results, and the search was on to find ever more effective chemicals for treating a variety of cancers.

In 1961, scientist Barnett Rosenberg (1926–) accidentally discovered that the metal platinum could be used to kill cancer cells. While studying electrical fields, Rosenberg found that bacteria stopped dividing altogether when he put them in an electric field he created. He was surprised to find that the bacteria were not reacting to the electric field but to being exposed to the platinum he had used to make the electric field. Eventually, Rosenberg and his colleagues created the platinum-based compound cisplatin for medical use. In 1978, the U.S. Food and Drug Administration (FDA) approved cisplatin for use in treating solid tumors. Platinum-based compounds are still used to treat ovarian cancer.

TEN GREAT QUESTIONS
TO ASK YOUR DOCTOR

1. What can I do to maintain good reproductive system health?

2. What should I do if I have swelling or feel pain in my pelvis?

3. When should I begin seeing a gynecologist?

4. How often should I visit the gynecologist?

5. What exams does the gynecologist do to check my ovaries?

6. What should I do if I have any itching, bleeding, or pain following my gynecologist exam?

7. Will a Pap smear tell the doctors anything about the condition of my ovaries?

8. If I get ovarian cancer, does it mean I won't be able to have children?

9. Does having ovarian cancer make me more vulnerable to other types of cancer?

10. Does my risk for ovarian cancer increase if my mother (sister/grandmother/aunt) was diagnosed with ovarian cancer?

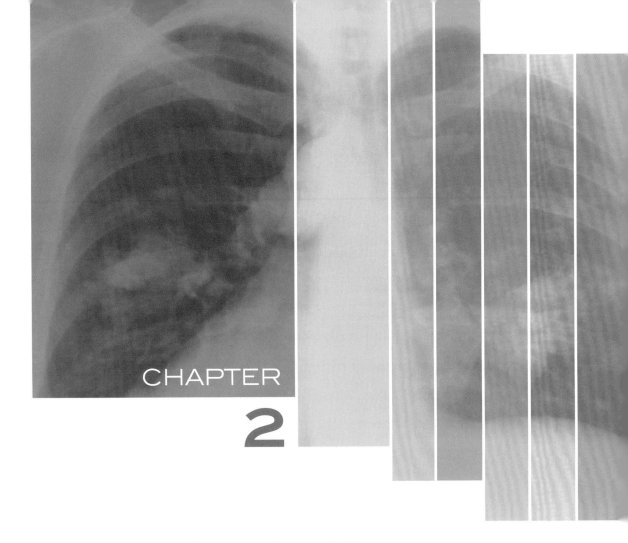

THE SCIENCE OF OVARIAN CANCER

Cancer occurs because something goes wrong with a gene that controls cell reproduction and growth. This chapter explains the changes that take place in genes that can result in cancer.

GENE MUTATIONS AND CANCER

Our genetic blueprint is carried in our chromosomes. These are tiny, threadlike strands of deoxyribonucleic acid (DNA) located in the nucleus (center) of all cells. Chromosomes are made up of genes, which

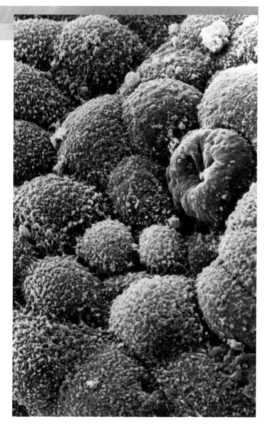

Pictured here are ovarian cancer cells, as seen through a scanning electron microscope. They are covered with tiny projections called microvilli and show the typical random arrangement of malignant cancer cells.

are specific sequences of DNA. Each gene controls the production of a particular protein, a basic building block of tissues and compounds in the body.

Your cells have two copies of every chromosome. One copy comes from your mother and one from your father. Sometimes, there is a defect, or mutation, in the copy of a gene that you received from one of your parents. There are two possible causes for this. Your parent could have inherited the defective gene from one of his or her parents and passed it on to you. Or, on the other hand, both of your parents could have normal versions of the gene, and your defective gene may have been the result of a mutation in one of your parents' sex cells (sperm and egg cells) that produced you. Either way, because these mutations came along with the genetic information you received from your parents, they are called inherited mutations.

MITOSIS, MEIOSIS, AND INHERITED MUTATIONS

Mitosis is the process by which most cells in the human body are replicated (copied). In mitosis, the chromosomes of a cell are copied to make a duplicate of each pair. Then, the cell divides into two identical "daughter cells." Sex cells, however, are made in a different process. Egg cells, produced in the female ovaries, and sperm cells, produced in the male testes, undergo a process of replication called meiosis. This involves two sets of cell division. The chromosomes in the sperm or egg cell mix together and then separate so that one pair of each type lines up at opposite ends of the cell. The cell then divides into two identical cells. Each of these two cells then undergoes meiosis. In this process, the chromosomes are not duplicated before they separate and line up at each end of the cells' nuclei. The cells then divide, forming four new cells. Each of these new cells has half the number of chromosomes (twenty-three) normally found in body cells. In sexual reproduction, the sperm and egg cells merge to form an embryo, which will have the full number of chromosomes (forty-six), having inherited one of each pair from its father and one of each pair from its mother.

Sometimes, when the chromosomes are copied during mitosis and meiosis, an error occurs in the sequence of DNA that makes up a gene. This change is called a mutation. A fertilized egg cell begins to divide, making many identical copies of genes in the original fertilized cell. Eventually, a complex series of chemical interactions causes these cells to develop into different types of tissue. As the weeks and months of pregnancy go by, the original mass of cells develops into an embryo, then a fetus, and finally into a baby. Because all the cells were copied from the original fertilized egg cell, they all have the same genes.

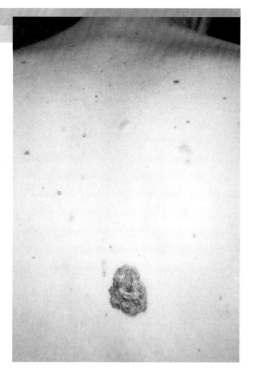

Not all cancer-causing gene mutations are inherited. The skin cancer shown here, a malignant melanoma, may be caused by mutations brought on by harmful exposure to the sun.

NON-INHERITED MUTATIONS

Not all gene mutations are inherited. Another type of mutation occurs when a healthy gene in your body is damaged because it is exposed to a toxic substance in the environment. This could be a pollutant, a chemical, or some kind of harmful radiation.

Finally, a mutation can occur accidentally when old cells in your body are copied to produce new cells. (All the cells in your body reproduce about fifty times during your life.) When a cell with a damaged gene reproduces, the damaged gene is copied along with all the other genes in that cell. All the daughter cells of the original cell will have the same mutation.

HOW MUTATIONS CAUSE CANCER

A mutation can cause a gene to work incorrectly or not at all. If this mutation affects the function of a gene that controls cell reproduction, then it can result in cancer. The fact that a person has a genetic mutation does not guarantee that he or she will get cancer; it merely increases the risk.

Genes that cause tumors are divided into two categories, depending on how they work: proto-oncogenes and tumor suppressor genes. Both types of genes can be inherited, and both can result from damage in the body.

PROTO-ONCOGENES

A proto-oncogene performs a useful function when it is intact, but it can become a cancer-causing gene if it is damaged. This type of gene generally produces a compound that controls cell growth. When the gene develops a mutation, however, it can become an oncogene (a gene that causes cancer). It can cause cancer in one of two ways: It can produce too much of a compound that makes cells reproduce, or it can make too little of a compound that stops them reproducing.

TUMOR SUPPRESSOR GENES

A tumor suppressor gene is a gene that stops cells reproducing. Sometimes, a tumor suppressor gene fails to work because of a mutation. In this case, other genes that cause cells to reproduce will keep doing so unchecked. As a result, cells keep reproducing, forming bigger and bigger masses of cells, or tumors.

THE TYPES OF OVARIAN CANCER

There are three main types of ovarian cancer: epithelial tumors, germ cell tumors, and stromal tumors.

EPITHELIAL CELL TUMORS

About 85–90 percent of ovarian cancer begins in the epithelial cells. Epithelial cell tumors grow from the tissue that lines or covers the ovaries. The word "tumor" is used to describe any group of cells that grows out

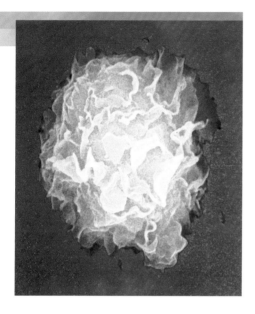

This is a colored picture of an epithelial ovarian cancer cell. It was taken with a scanning electron microscope, which scans the cell in tiny increments to build up a 3-D image.

of control, forming a lump or mass of cells. Not all tumors are cancerous. Only a tumor that spreads and creates new tumors is cancerous. Tumors that form a mass but do not spread are called benign tumors. These tumors may cause pain. Also, if they grow large enough, they may block fluid from passing through an organ, or they may press on nearby nerves and organs. Therefore, it may be necessary to remove them. Benign tumors do not invade other organs and are therefore unlikely to result in death.

Cancerous tumors, in contrast, do invade other organs. If they interfere with the function of critical organs such as the liver or lungs, then they can result in death. These cancerous tumors are called malignant tumors.

There are four types of epithelial tumors: serous, mucinous, endometrioid, and clear cell tumors. Serous tumors can be benign, malignant, or borderline. The majority of serous tumors are benign and often fluid-filled. That is why they are called serous, which comes from the word "serum," the clear fluid part of the blood. The usual treatment is to remove the ovary that contains the tumor. About 30 percent of epithelial tumors are malignant. These make up 85–90 percent of malignant ovarian tumors. The cells of borderline tumors have some of the characteristics of cancer cells, but they rarely spread and are rarely fatal. They occur primarily in women thirty to fifty years of age. This is different from other types of ovarian tumors, which occur primarily in women from forty to seventy-nine years of age. Mucinous tumors are similar to serous tumors. About 80 percent of them are benign.

Most epithelial tumors grow from the epithelial cells lining and covering the ovary. A small number grow from other epithelial tissue such as the tissue lining the uterus. The lining of the uterus is called the endometrium. When epithelial cancer grows from endometrial tissue, the tumor is an endometrioid tumor. Clear cell tumors also grow mainly from endometrial tissue. They have large bodies filled with clear cytoplasm (the fluid that fills the body of a cell), which gives these tumors their name.

GERM CELL TUMORS

Germ cell tumors grow from the cells that produce eggs. About 5 percent of ovarian cancers are germ cell tumors. Most germ cell tumors are benign. However, a small number are malignant. The most common type of germ cell tumor is called a teratoma. This type of tumor typically occurs in women younger than fifty years of age. The most common type is the mature teratoma. It can occur as a solid tumor or as a cyst— a fluid-filled, sac-like growth. Mature teratomas frequently contain recognizable tissues such as hair, bone, and teeth. They are usually benign and are treated by removing the ovary. Immature teratomas occur mostly in girls under the age of eighteen. They contain cells that resemble lung, brain, or connective tissue cells. The exact cause of germ cell tumors is not known. Researchers believe they grow from germ cells that failed to reach their proper place in the ovaries when the female fetus was developing. These misplaced germ cells may then divide and develop the characteristics of specific types of tissue.

There are two other types of germ cell cancer, but they are very rare. They primarily affect young women in their teens and twenties.

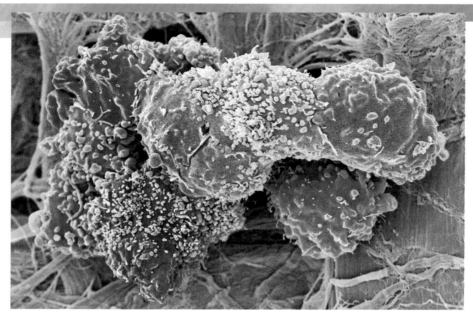

This is a colored scanning electron microscope image of teratoma cancer cells. Teratomas grow from sperm and egg cells.

Dysgerminomas are a slow-growing type of cancer that is malignant. This grows so slowly that 75 percent of women who have it are cured by surgery alone. Another 15 percent are cured with a combination of surgery and chemotherapy. Yolk sac tumors, which start in the ovary, grow quickly but are quite responsive to chemotherapy.

STROMAL TUMORS
Stromal tumors make up about 5–7 percent of ovarian cancer cases. These tumors grow from the connective tissue that attaches the ovaries to the pelvic wall. Most stromal tumors affect women over the age of fifty. However, younger girls account for about 5 percent of the cases. As with other types of ovarian cancer, stromal tumors can be either benign or malignant.

Stromal tumors produce estrogen and progesterone, two hormones important in the development of female sex characteristics. As a result, these tumors in a young girl can cause symptoms of puberty to occur prematurely. Rarely, stromal tumors produce male sex hormones, rather than female ones. In this case, a girl or woman may start to show male sexual characteristics. For example, she may grow facial hair or stop menstruating.

OVULATION AND OVARIAN CANCER

The older a female is, the greater her risk of ovarian cancer. Most cases of ovarian cancer occur in women between the ages of forty and seventy-nine, with incidence peaking around the late seventies. Outside of genetic factors and age, ovulation is a key risk factor for ovarian cancer. In general, the more times a woman ovulates in her life, the greater her risk of ovarian cancer. For this reason, ovarian cancer occurs more frequently in women who have never been pregnant, breastfed a baby, or taken birth control pills (all of which cause ovulation to stop for a while).

Ovarian cancer is more likely to occur in women who start menstruating at a very young age (earlier than twelve) or stop getting their period much later than the average age (significantly after fifty). The increased risk may be related to the production of the hormone progesterone.

GENETIC RISK FACTORS

Researchers have linked ovarian cancer to mutations of two specific genes: BRCA1 and BRCA2. BRCA1 is located on chromosome 17, and BRCA2 is located on chromosome 13. BRCA1 and BRCA2 are tumor suppressor genes. One of the things that tumor suppressor genes do is keep cells from growing out of control. If one of these genes mutates, then it may no longer be able to perform this function, leading to the growth of tumors. It is now possible to perform genetic testing for mutations of the BRCA1 and BRCA2 genes.

The risk of ovarian cancer also increases if a female has a type of colon cancer called hereditary nonpolyposis colon cancer (HNPCC). HNPCC is caused by a mutation in any one of several genes that are responsible for correcting mistakes in DNA when it is copied to produce new cells. If these genes fail to function because of a mutation, then "mistakes" may go uncorrected in genes responsible for cell growth or in tumor suppressor genes. Mutations in these genes can lead to colon cancer and to ovarian cancer as well.

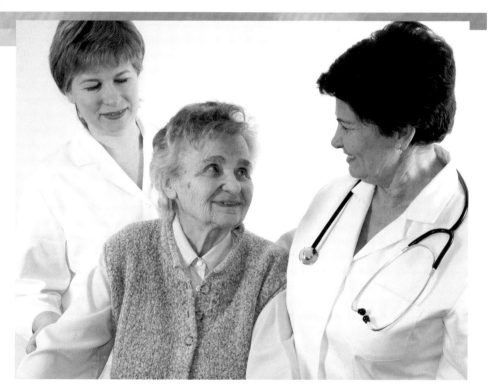

Ovarian cancer mainly affects older women, and the risk of ovarian cancer increases with age.

MYTHS AND FACTS

MYTH Ovarian cysts often develop into ovarian cancer.

FACT Some ovarian cysts can be cancerous. However, ovarian cysts—which are quite common—are usually benign (harmless) and go away on their own.

MYTH It's impossible to predict who may get ovarian cancer.

FACT Several risk factors for this disease have been identified. They include early menstruation; increasing age; mutations of the BRCA-1 and BRCA-2 genes; family history of ovarian, breast, or colorectal cancer; personal history of breast cancer; and never bearing a child or having a child later in life.

MYTH There is no cure for ovarian cancer.

FACT Ovarian cancer used to be a very dire diagnosis. However, advances in diagnostic technology and medical treatment have greatly increased survival rates. Close to 90 percent of the women whose ovarian cancer is detected early and treated properly survive for at least five years.

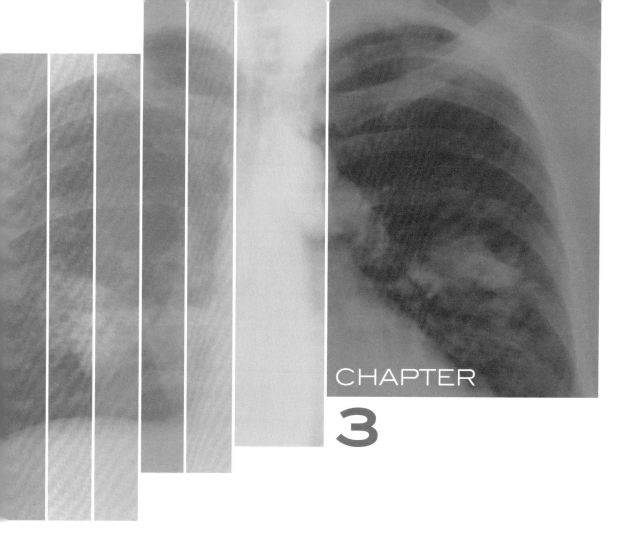

DETECTION AND TREATMENT

This chapter explains how doctors diagnose ovarian cancer and how it is treated once it has been found.

DIAGNOSING OVARIAN CANCER

The most notable sign of ovarian cancer is swelling in the abdomen. This happens because fluid accumulates, causing the abdomen to bulge out. In rare cases, abnormal bleeding between periods may occur. Other signs include abdominal or pelvic pain, a frequent urge to urinate, and digestion problems. In some cases, a doctor may find something abnormal during a routine pelvic exam.

There is no standard, reliable test to detect ovarian cancer that is suitable for screening large numbers of women. However, there are tests that can be performed if a woman has a family history of ovarian or colon cancer. The tests are also used if a woman has possible cancer symptoms or if her doctor finds something abnormal during a routine pelvic exam.

SCANNING FOR TUMORS

If the doctor detects symptoms that indicate an ovarian growth, then he or she may order an imaging test. Most ovarian growths turn out to be cysts or benign tumors, so being sent for an imaging test is not necessarily a bad sign.

One common imaging method is ultrasound. In this type of test, a technician runs a handheld device over the woman's abdomen. The device generates sound waves, which bounce off the internal organs. A computer interprets the signals

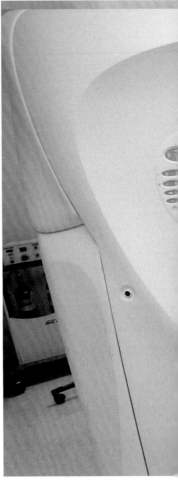

and produces an image on a monitor, showing what the ovaries and other nearby organs look like. If there is a tumor in the ovaries, then it usually will be visible in the picture.

If the results of the ultrasound indicate the possibility of a tumor, then the patient may be sent for an additional scan called magnetic resonance imaging (MRI). In this test, the patient lies in a large machine, which uses high-powered magnets and radio waves to create a series of pictures of the internal organs. MRI allows the doctor to see the exact

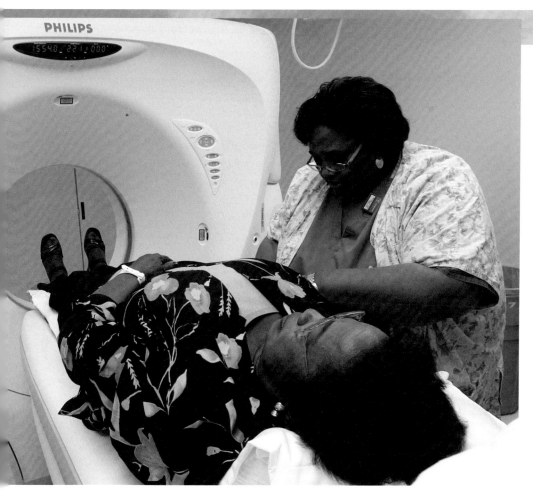

In this photo, a cancer patient is being prepared for a CT scan. Modern scanning technologies allow doctors to find out more about tumors without having to cut into the patient.

location, size, and shape of the tumor. Computed tomography (CT) is yet another type of scan used to create a picture of the inside of the body. CT scans are similar to MRIs, but they use X-rays instead of radio waves to create an image.

OTHER TESTS FOR OVARIAN CANCER

In a laparoscopy, a tube with a tiny camera is inserted through a small abdominal incision. The picture from the camera is displayed on a monitor. Laparoscopy allows the doctor to directly see the ovaries and surrounding areas.

The doctor may also have a blood test done for a tumor marker. A tumor marker is a substance that is produced by tumors or by non-tumor cells in response to the presence of a tumor. In the case of ovarian cancer, the tumor puts out an antigen called C125. Antigens are substances in the blood that cause a reaction in a person's immune system. If there is an elevated amount of the C125 antigen in a woman's blood, then it is a sign that she may have ovarian cancer.

If there is evidence of ovarian cancer from these tests or from the scans, then the doctor may have additional tests performed to see if the cancer has spread to other organs or parts of the body. Other tests might include:

— **Barium enema X-rays**, in which a chalky liquid is inserted into the colon to make the colon show up on X-rays. This tells the doctor whether any cancer has spread to the colon.
— **A colonoscopy**, in which a tube with a tiny camera is inserted through the anus into the colon to allow the doctor to see if there is any cancer in the colon.
— **A chest X-ray**, to see if the cancer has spread to the lungs.

If the doctor sees anything that might be cancer during these tests, then he or she may perform a biopsy. For this procedure, a small piece of tissue is removed from the suspected tumor. The tissue is then examined under a microscope in a lab to see if it contains cancer cells.

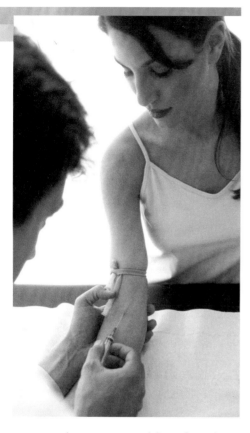

A blood sample is all that is needed for some genetic tests. The genes in the nuclei of blood cells carry the mutation that the tests look for.

GENETIC TESTING

Genetic tests can identify some of the mutations that increase the risk of ovarian cancer. For instance, there is a test for the BRCA1 and BRCA2 mutations. Most women who undergo genetic testing do so simply to get a better understanding of their cancer risks. However, some women who test positive for these types of mutations elect to have their ovaries and fallopian tubes surgically removed. (This is more likely if they are beyond childbearing age.) It is important to note that not every woman who has such mutations will develop the disease, and not all cases of ovarian cancer are hereditary.

THE STAGES OF OVARIAN CANCER

Doctors identify the severity of ovarian cancer by dividing it into stages and substages. Stage 1 means that the cancer is only affecting the ovaries. Stage 2 ovarian cancer is affecting the ovaries and other reproductive organs, such as the fallopian tubes or the uterus. Stage 2 ovarian cancer may also affect other pelvic organs, like the bladder, but it has not spread beyond the pelvic area. In stage 3 ovarian cancer, the cancer has spread into the abdomen or into the lymph nodes. The lymph nodes are glands that produce immune system cells. Lymph glands are concentrated in the neck, armpits, and groin and under the uterus. In stage 4 ovarian cancer, the cancer has spread to other organs, such as the lungs or liver. Stages are further subdivided into three levels, A, B, and C, which indicate increasing severity.

Cancer is identified by the organ in which it originated, not by the organ where it is found. So, even when ovarian cancer spreads to other organs, it is still considered ovarian cancer.

TREATMENTS FOR OVARIAN CANCER

The most common treatments for ovarian cancer are surgery and chemotherapy. At times, radiation therapy is also used.

SURGERY

Treatment for ovarian cancer usually involves surgical removal of the affected ovary and often other reproductive organs as well. If the ovarian cancer is caught in an early stage, then the doctor may simply remove the affected ovary. However, if the cancer is advanced, then the surgeon will generally remove both of the ovaries, the uterus, and the fallopian tubes. In severe cases of ovarian cancer, surgery is often combined with chemotherapy.

CHEMOTHERAPY

In chemotherapy, or chemo, a patient is given strong drugs that kill fast-growing cancer cells. Chemotherapy drugs are usually given intravenously—delivered through a needle inserted into a vein.

Sometimes, however, the drugs are delivered directly into the abdomen. According to the American Cancer Society, studies have shown that using both methods can improve a woman's chances of surviving ovarian cancer.

Chemotherapy is most often used after surgery if the cancer has progressed to stage 1C or if the cancer is stage 2, 3, or 4. Chemotherapy is common if the cancer comes back after treatment. A chemotherapy treatment can take several hours and is usually given once every three to four weeks. It's usual to have six to twelve treatments. Chemotherapy drugs work in one of two ways: either by killing

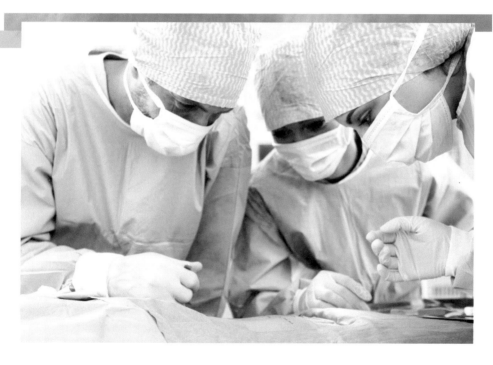

Surgery is usually necessary to treat ovarian cancer. How extensive the surgery is depends on the stage of the cancer, as well as which organs are affected.

cancer cells, or by keeping cancer cells from reproducing. Frequently, a combination of chemotherapy drugs is given so that both of these approaches are used at the same time.

Platinum-based drugs, like cisplatin or carboplatin, have been found to be effective against ovarian cancer. They are given in chemotherapy either by themselves or in combination with other drugs such as Taxol that also inhibit cell growth and division.

RADIATION

Radiation therapy is most often used to treat ovarian cancer that has spread from the ovaries to other reproductive and/or pelvic organs but has not spread to the abdomen or other organs. The goal is to kill any cancer that is left after surgery. Radiation is also used along with surgery and chemotherapy to treat advanced ovarian cancer. The goal is to shrink tumors so that the patient suffers less.

The radiation is usually delivered by a machine that emits powerful X-rays that are aimed at the area where the cancer occurred. Sometimes, however, radioactive rods or pellets may be implanted in the abdomen to focus the radiation at a key spot. Treatment usually takes only a few minutes. Radiation therapy treatments are usually given for several days in a row every week for several weeks. The technician will deliver the radiation to specific points on the patient's body, protecting the rest of her body from exposure as much as possible.

SIDE EFFECTS OF RADIATION AND CHEMOTHERAPY

Chemotherapy and radiation do have some negative side effects. Chemotherapy kills fast-growing cancer cells, but it also kills fast-growing normal cells, including the cells that line the stomach. For this reason, chemotherapy often results in digestion problems, nausea, and vomiting.

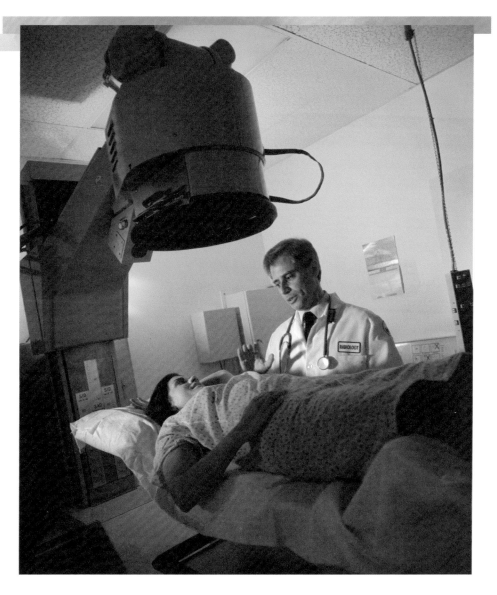

This woman is receiving radiation therapy. Before starting the treatment, the doctor isolates the area to be treated and marks spots on the patient's body to pinpoint the areas to be irradiated.

COMPLEMENTARY TREATMENTS

Complementary treatments are techniques that are not part of conventional medical treatment. When used alone, these therapies are not effective in curing cancer. However, they have been shown to be helpful to some cancer patients when combined with conventional treatment. Many of these treatments help patients by relieving symptoms of the disease and side effects of treatment. They also reduce stress, which helps the body to heal itself. Examples of complementary treatments include:

- **Massage therapy:** Massage therapy should be performed by a licensed massage therapist. It can help relieve muscle spasms and, thus, reduce pain as well as provide relaxation.
- **Acupuncture:** Acupuncture is a traditional Chinese therapy in which thin needles are inserted at key points in the body. Some people find that acupuncture can help with symptoms of nausea and pain.
- **Meditation:** Meditation is a method of calming the mind and body that can reduce stress and help the body to relax.
- **Herbal supplements:** Many plants have natural chemicals that have a variety of effects just like conventional medications. Their effects include relaxing the body, improving one's mood, helping one get to sleep, improving immune function, treating constipation, and others. However, herbal supplements are still medicines, even though they are natural ones.

- **High-dose vitamins:** Vitamins are necessary for the healthy functioning of the body. For example, vitamin E helps to build up blood cells, the B vitamins are necessary for healthy muscles and nerve function, and vitamin A is necessary for healthy skin, bones, and mucous membranes. Some people believe that taking large doses of vitamins helps to protect the body. However, many vitamins are dangerous if they are taken in too great a dose.

- **Nutrition:** There are many popular books on the use of proper nutrition to treat various ailments. Many such nutritional approaches emphasize eating fruits and vegetables, which are high in vitamins and low in fat. It makes sense that eating a well-balanced, healthy diet low in fat will make you feel better and will better equip your body to withstand treatment. However, cancer cannot be cured by eating any particular food.

- **Imagery:** Imagery techniques involve focusing the mind so that it influences your body to fight the cancer. Imaging can involve picturing a positive result for treatment, picturing the cancer being destroyed, picturing yourself in a pleasant location to relax your body, and other techniques. These techniques are similar to those used by athletes who picture themselves winning in order to improve their performance. Although there is no evidence that imagery techniques help cure cancer, they can help to improve the symptoms through relaxation and reducing stress.

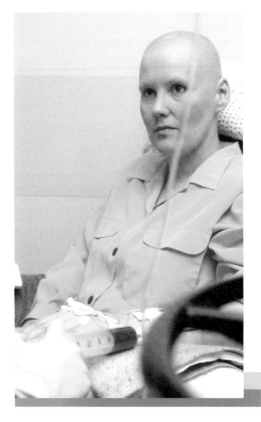

This young woman is receiving chemotherapy. The medications are given intravenously—in a solution that is dripped into a vein through a needle inserted into her arm.

Hair follicles, too, are fast-growing cells, so hair loss is another side effect of chemotherapy. However, in most cases, the hair loss is temporary, and the hair grows back once treatment has been completed and the chemotherapy drugs are out of the patient's system. Other side effects from radiation and chemotherapy treatments include constipation or diarrhea and fatigue. Doctors can prescribe medications to help with these problems.

Both chemotherapy and radiation can reduce the number of white blood cells, which help the body fight off infection. Therefore, chemo and radiation patients may get sick more easily. Chemotherapy and radiation may also affect other components of the blood. For example, they may reduce the number of red blood cells, resulting in anemia, which can increase the feeling of fatigue. Chemotherapy may also reduce the platelet count in blood. Platelets are sticky elements that help blood to clot and form scabs. People undergoing chemotherapy or radiation treatment may bleed more easily from injuries, and it may take the bleeding a longer time than normal to stop.

Finally, chemotherapy can affect the nerves that run down your spinal cord into other parts of your body. The most common effects are tingling or numbness in the hands and feet.

CHECKING ON RECOVERY

During treatment, the doctor will check on the patient's progress through regular testing. If the patient had evidence of C125 in her blood prior to treatment, then the doctor may use a blood test for this antigen to see if the level is decreasing. Also, the doctor may use scanning to check on the progress of treatment. Even if the cancer appears to be completely gone, the doctor will most likely have the patient undergo testing periodically to verify that it has not come back.

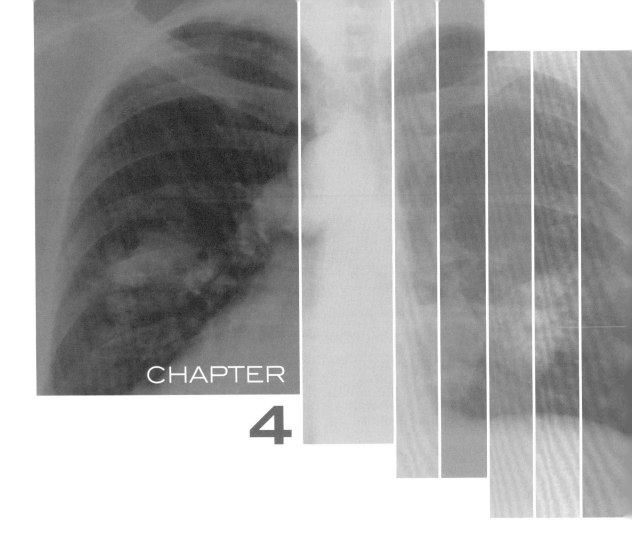

CHAPTER

4

LIVING WITH OVARIAN CANCER

Finding out that one has cancer can be a shocking and upsetting experience. There are many issues that have to be dealt with. There are both short-term and long-term issues that relate to living with cancer. Patients may feel tired and weak, not only from the cancer itself but also from the stress of treatment. For this reason, it is important for cancer patients to try to get adequate rest and to not overdo things. It is just as important for them to get adequate nutrition in order to maintain their strength and to allow their bodies to build new tissue. In addition, it is important for patients to get plenty of sleep and to get some exercise—without overdoing it. Exercise helps keep the body strong, and it can also help in reducing stress.

RECOVERY AND FERTILITY

One area that is usually of concern to women with ovarian cancer is their future ability to have children. Whether or not a woman can have children after surgery depends on the type of ovarian cancer and how advanced it was. If a woman is of childbearing age and the cancer is caught early, then the doctor may elect to remove only the ovary with the tumor and the fallopian tube on the same side. That way, the woman can still have children with the eggs produced by the other ovary. If the cancer is in both ovaries, then the doctor may remove both ovaries but leave the uterus, so that the woman has the option of having a child using donor eggs. In that case, the eggs from another woman (the

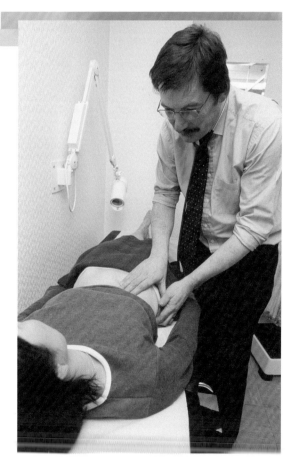

Here, a doctor checks the abdomen of a patient. Regular checkups are important after treatment for cancer to ensure that any signs of the cancer coming back are caught early.

donor) are fertilized in a laboratory and are then implanted into the woman's uterus. If the ovarian cancer is advanced, then the surgeon will often remove both ovaries, the uterus, and the fallopian tubes. After such surgery, it would not be possible for the woman to bear children.

COPING WITH CANCER IN THE FAMILY

If someone in your family has cancer, then there are several things that you should know. First, if a parent, sibling, or other relative you are close to becomes seriously ill, then it is easy to feel that somehow it is your fault. This is especially true if relations have been strained or if you have been having arguments. However, you should understand that you are not responsible for that person getting cancer. Cancer is caused by a random genetic mutation, and nothing you did or did not do could have had any effect. Second, if someone you care about has cancer, then you may feel angry and frightened. This is especially true if the person involved is your mother. You rely on her for both emotional and practical support. At the same time, you may feel that you shouldn't "act like a baby" or worry her by talking about your feelings. Understand that adults have exactly the same feelings of anger and fear. These feelings are normal. Talk to your friends, a counselor, or a support group about your feelings. Also be aware that if your mother is ill, then your father may have exactly the same feelings of fear that you do. Worrying may make him short-tempered and impatient at times. Understand that he is not "on your case" because he blames you or doesn't care about you.

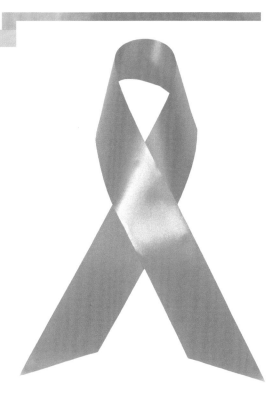

A teal ribbon is the symbol of ovarian cancer awareness. Survivors and supporters wear the ribbons to show support for research and education on ovarian cancer.

EMOTIONAL SUPPORT

Dealing with ovarian cancer can be scary and stressful. Diagnosis, treatment, and recovery from the disease all raise their own issues. Having cancer, as well as experiencing the changes in one's body from treatment, can affect how one feels about oneself. Cancer patients may also feel self-conscious about how others see them. They may also be fearful that the cancer will come back. Because of these types of mental stress, it is sometimes a good idea to talk to a mental health professional or counselor who works with cancer patients and their families.

Counseling, however, is not the only option. There is also a variety of support groups for people who are being treated for cancer and for their families. If your mother or someone else close to you has cancer, then you may want to join such a group. The families of cancer patients often need help coping just as much as the patient does. Support groups offer a chance to share your feelings with others who understand what you're going through, in a more informal setting.

In addition to emotional support, such groups can also provide tips on coping with the effects of the disease and treatment. Lists of support groups can be found on the Web sites of reputable organizations such as the American Cancer Society (www.cancer.org), as well as through recommendations at the facility where you or your family member is undergoing cancer treatment.

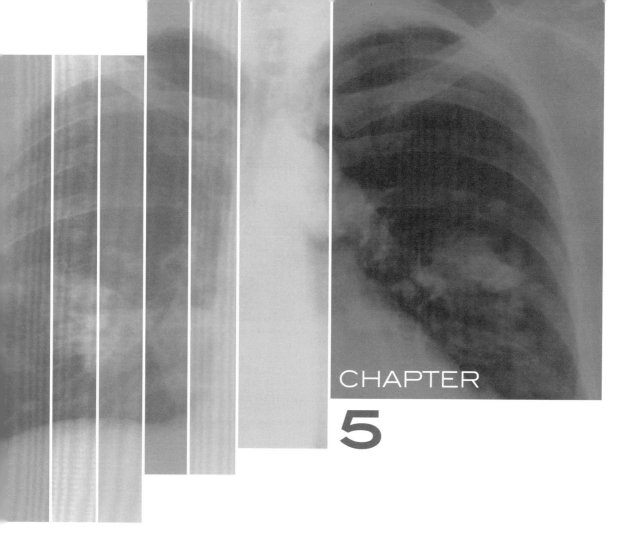

NEW FRONTIERS

Ovarian cancer is the result of a genetic defect. Therefore, much of the experimental research being undertaken uses genes to discover the causes of and treatments for ovarian cancer. This chapter examines some of the experimental techniques on the horizon.

FINDING THE OVARIAN CANCER GENES

A key to catching ovarian cancer early and treating it is identifying the genes responsible for it. Some genes that increase the risk of ovarian cancer have already been found, like BRCA1 and BRCA2, as discussed in chapter 2. However, there is much that we still don't know about which genes cause the various types of ovarian cancer. Therefore, one area of research is aimed at discovering more genes responsible for specific types of ovarian cancer.

For example, in 2005, researchers at the Johns Hopkins University Kimmel Cancer Research Center in Baltimore, Maryland, identified a gene that is responsible for one of the most aggressive forms of ovarian cancer. The gene is called Rsf-1. Researchers identified an increased amount of Rsf-1 in ovarian cancer by studying the entire genome (all of the genes) of seven different cell lines of ovarian cancer. A cell line is a group of cells grown from one particular cell. The researchers found that much larger numbers of this gene were present in several of the cell lines. Identifying genes such as Rsf-1 could someday lead to the development of a test that looks for abnormally high levels of such genes. A test like this one could ultimately help to identify the presence of ovarian cancer much earlier, when treatment is more likely to be successful.

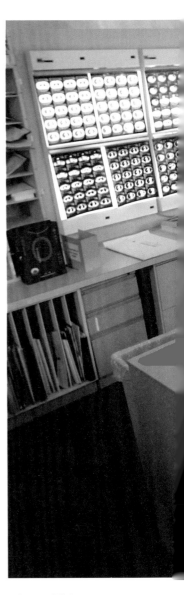

WHAT IS GENE THERAPY?

In the past two decades, scientists have developed new tools that allow them to alter genes. The process of modifying genes is called genetic engineering. Gene therapy uses genetic engineering techniques to replace genes that don't work with new ones that do.

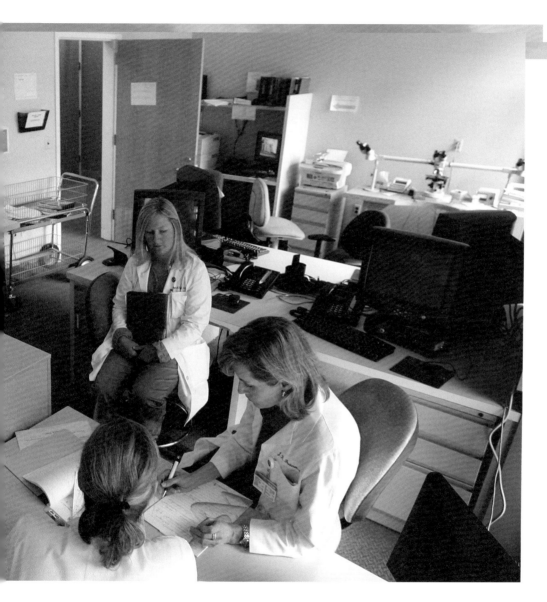

Researchers at the Johns Hopkins University Kimmel Cancer Research Center examine results from patients. The center is working to develop a better understanding of ovarian and other cancers.

CLINICAL TRIALS

Many new approaches are being investigated to treat ovarian cancer. These treatments have not yet been proven effective and safe. If conventional treatment has not cured the cancer, or if the cancer returns after treatment and conventional treatment does not help, then the patient may choose to participate in a clinical trial. This is a test of a new therapy to establish if it works and is safe. Clinical trials test such treatments on volunteers. The tests are overseen by government agencies such as the National Institutes of Health (NIH)

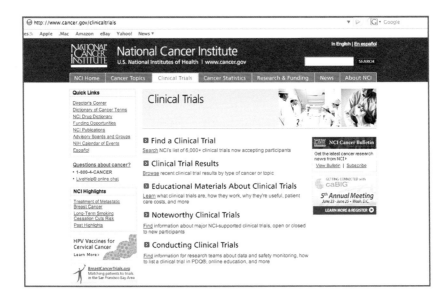

The U. S. National Cancer Institute maintains a Web site (www.cancer.gov) where you can learn about the latest clinical trials that are being conducted and their results.

and the U.S. Food and Drug Administration (FDA). Clinical trials may be testing better versions of treatments already in use. For example, they may test new combinations of chemotherapy drugs, which researchers hope will be more effective. On the other hand, clinical trials may test entirely new approaches to treating ovarian cancer, like gene therapy.

Participating in a clinical trial involves many risks. The treatment may not work, or it may have unpleasant side effects. Sometimes, however, people who have an otherwise incurable problem feel that it is worth trying a therapy that has even a small chance of succeeding. In addition, even though the treatment may not work, some people feel that by participating, they are helping with research that may save lives in the future and, thus, are doing something worthwhile.

Information on clinical trials can be obtained from the Web sites of organizations such as the American Cancer Society (www.cancer.org), the National Cancer Institute (www.cancer.gov), and the Food and Drug Administration (www.fda.gov).

Gene therapy is in the very early stages, and treatments are still experimental. However, scientists around the world are working on new gene-based solutions to a wide range of diseases, including cancer.

Scientists can alter genes using several different methods:

- They can repair a gene by replacing the defective part with a correct segment.
- They can remove a gene that is not working and insert a new working gene in its place.

They can turn a gene that controls a cancer gene on or off. For example, turning on a tumor suppressor gene could cause it to turn off a cancer-causing gene that is allowing cells to grow out of control.

HOW GENE THERAPY WORKS

The basis of gene therapy is replacing genes that don't work with ones that do. Periodically, cells replicate and divide to make new cells. During this process, the cell's genes are copied. If a new gene is inserted into

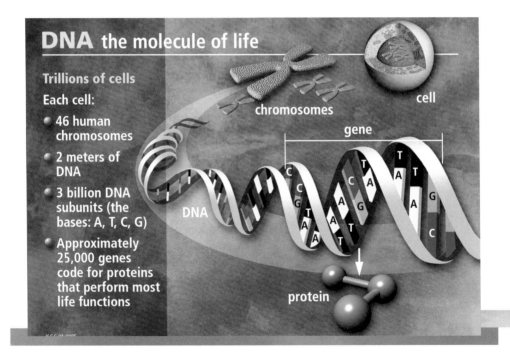

DNA the molecule of life

Trillions of cells

Each cell:

- **46 human chromosomes**
- **2 meters of DNA**
- **3 billion DNA subunits (the bases: A, T, C, G)**
- **Approximately 25,000 genes code for proteins that perform most life functions**

chromosomes

cell

gene

DNA

protein

This illustration shows a gene—a segment of DNA. The order of the nucleotides (A, T, C, and G) tells a cell how to make a specific protein. Gene therapy attempts to correct the order of nucleotides in a defective gene.

a cell that divides, then a copy of this new gene will be present in both cells that result.

The key to gene therapy is getting the new gene into the cell. The difficulty is that the chromosomes, which contain the genes, are located in the nucleus of the cell, which is surrounded by a membrane. Scientists have known for a long time that viruses can get through the membrane of a cell in order to inject their own DNA into the cell. (This is how viruses cause infection.) Therefore, scientists often use viruses as a means to deliver genes to cells. First, they render the virus unable to cause infection. Next, they insert a new gene into the virus DNA. A solution containing the genetically engineered viruses is then infused into the patient's body through a vein. The viruses are carried through the patient's blood to cells. The viruses then "infect" the target cells with the new gene. When the cells reproduce, the new gene will be copied along with the rest of their DNA.

GENE THERAPY FOR OVARIAN CANCER

One of the genes commonly found to be involved in ovarian cancer is called p53. It is a gene that causes cells to die at the appropriate time. Mutations in p53 cause cells to live longer than they should. When new cells grow together with the old cells that normally should have died, a tumor often develops. Many current clinical trials are looking for an effective way to deliver healthy p53 to ovarian cancer cells. Results have been promising in studies in which ovarian cancer cells in laboratories were infected with viruses carrying a correct copy of the gene. Cells did take up the gene, and there was evidence that the gene worked. This p53 therapy is in its early stages, and much work remains to be done to find a way to deliver the gene successfully in human subjects.

Another approach to treating ovarian tumors is being investigated by researchers at the Pittsburgh School of Medicine. In 2006, a team led

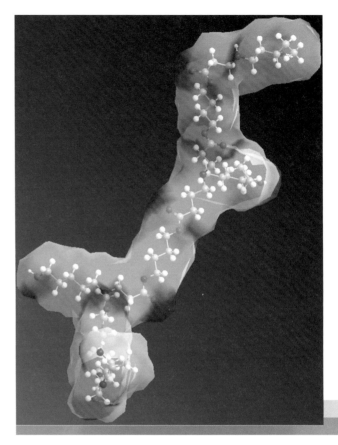

This illustration shows part of a polymer developed at the Massachusetts Institute of Technology. The polymer has been shown to be as effective as viruses for delivering genes to cells.

by Dr. David L. Bartlett demonstrated a gene therapy–based vaccine against ovarian cancer. The researchers performed a study using mice that had been infected with ovarian cancer cells. They then used a virus to deliver a "suicide" gene to the cancer cells. This special gene causes the cancer cells to produce a toxic compound that kills them. The gene therapy successfully kept tumors from growing in all the treated mice. In contrast, tumors grew in all the untreated mice.

One of the problems with gene therapy stems from the use of viruses as delivery mechanisms. Even though they cannot cause infection in the person receiving them, viruses can still cause an allergic reaction. This can happen because a person's immune system cells may recognize the viruses as foreign particles and attack them. Some allergic reactions are mild, but some are very serious and can even be life threatening. To solve the virus problem, researchers at the Cancer Research Center at the Massachusetts Institute of Technology (MIT) are working on designing a new delivery mechanism for genes. They have developed a polymer that can be used to deliver genes. A polymer is a human-made compound composed of many linked molecules. Plastics, for example, are polymers. The MIT researchers have successfully used their polymer to deliver genes to mice with ovarian cancer. The polymer is relatively inexpensive and breaks down to harmless by-products in the body after delivering the genes. The polymer can be targeted to specific cells, which is critical for treating cancer.

Modern science and technology are being used to constantly improve therapies for treating ovarian cancer. And, as time goes on, there is little doubt that better detection methods and new treatments will be developed to treat this disease.

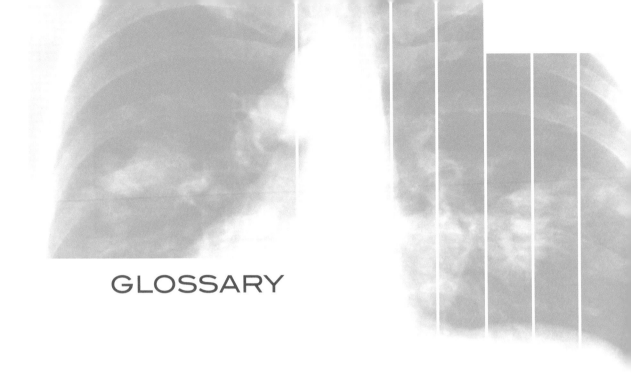

GLOSSARY

abdomen Area of the body below the stomach.

antigen Substance that causes an immune system reaction.

benign tumor Non-cancerous tumor that doesn't spread.

chromosome Threadlike strands of DNA that carry our genetic blueprint.

cisplatin Platinum-based compound that is used to treat ovarian cancer.

connective tissue Tissue that supports and connects body parts.

cortex Main part of an ovary, where eggs are produced.

cytoplasm Fluid that fills the main body of a cell.

deoxyribonucleic acid (DNA) Material that makes up chromosomes.

electron Basic particle, one of the components of an atom; it produces an electric charge.

epithelial cell Type of cell that lines the internal and external surfaces of the body and its organs.

fallopian tubes Tubes that run from the ovaries to the uterus, through which an egg travels when released by an ovary.

follicle Structure in an ovary that releases an egg.

gene Sequence of DNA on a chromosome; it carries the code for a protein.

germinal epithelium Outer layer of the ovary.

intravenous Inserted into the body through a needle placed in a vein.

lymph Fluid in which immune system cells circulate.

malignant Cancerous tumor that spreads to other organs.

medulla Innermost part of the ovary.

meiosis Process in which sperm and egg cells are formed.

menstruation Monthly shedding of the uterine lining (also called a woman's period).

metastasis Spreading of cancer from where it starts to other parts of the body.

microvilli Tiny, finger-like projections on the surface of a cell.

mitosis Process in which chromosomes are duplicated and two new cells are formed.

mutation Change or alteration in a gene.

ovulation Releasing of an egg by an ovary.

parasite Organism that feeds on the body.

placenta Organ that provides nutrition to a baby in the womb.

platinum Grayish-white metal.

puberty Age at which a person becomes capable of reproduction.

scanning electron microscope Type of microscope in which the tissue to be scanned is passed through a beam of electrons to create a 3-D image.

spontaneously Appearing suddenly without warning.

tumor Abnormal mass of cells.

vein Blood vessel that carries blood back to the heart.

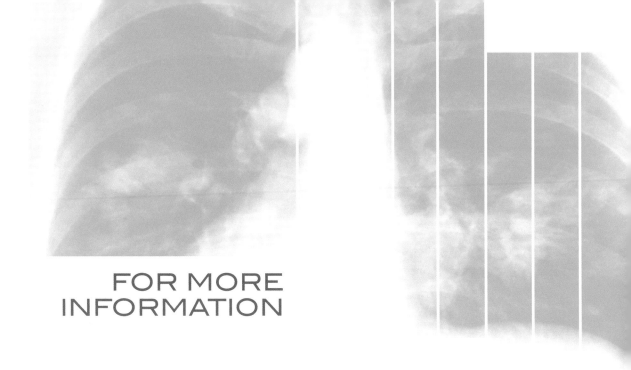

FOR MORE
INFORMATION

American Cancer Society
1599 Clifton Road NE
Atlanta, GA 30329
(800) ACS-2345 (227-2345)
Web site: http://www.cancer.org
The American Cancer Society is a nationwide, community-based
    voluntary health organization with more than 3,400 local offices.
    It provides helpful information on cancer via publications, an
    informative Web site, and by phone.

American Institute of Cancer Research
1759 R Street NW
Washington, DC 2009
(202) 328-7226
Web site: http://www.aicr.org
This organization provides the latest information on cancer research
    and offers a variety of printed resources on cancer.

Canadian Cancer Society
10 Alcorn Avenue, Suite 2000
Toronto, ON M4V 3B1
Canada
(416) 961-7223
Web site: http://www.cancer.ca
This site provides the latest news on cancer in Canada and information
    on specific types of cancer.

Kids Konnected
27071 Cabot Road, Suite 102
Laguna, CA 92653
(949) 582-5443
Web site: http://www.kidskonnected.org
This organization, supported by many major corporations, is devoted
    to supporting kids who have a parent with cancer or have lost a
    parent to it. It has separate resources for children and teenagers,
    including camps, support groups, and a Web site.

National Ovarian Cancer Coalition
500 NE Spanish River Boulevard, Suite 8
Boca Raton, FL 33431
(561) 393-7275
Web site: http://www.ovarian.org
The mission of this organization is to raise awareness and promote
    education about ovarian cancer.

Ovarian Cancer National Alliance
910 17th Street NW, Suite 1190
Washington, DC 20006

(212) 331-1332
Web site: http://www.ovariancancer.org
This organization provides resources for ovarian cancer patients,
    including newsletters.

WEB SITES

Due to the changing nature of Internet links, Rosen Publishing has
developed an online list of Web sites related to the subject of this book.
This site is updated regularly. Please use this link to access the list:

http://www.rosenlinks.com/cms/ovar

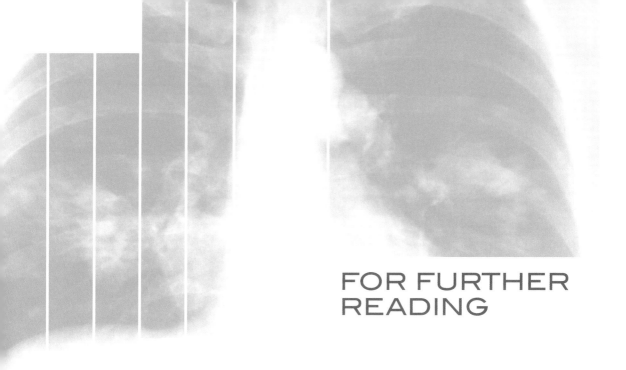

FOR FURTHER READING

Caldwell, Wilma A., ed. *Cancer Information for Teens: Health Tips About Cancer Awareness, Prevention, Diagnosis, and Treatment.* Detroit, MI: Omnigraphics, 2004.

Dizon, Don S. *100 Questions and Answers About Ovarian Cancer.* Boston, MA: Jones and Bartlett, 2006.

Feuerstein, Michael, and Patricia Findley. *The Cancer Survivor's Guide: The Essential Handbook to Life After Cancer.* New York, NY: Marlowe & Co., 2006.

Matray-devoti, Judy. *Cancer Drugs.* New York, NY: Chelsea House, 2005.

Miron, Ayala. *Ovarian Cancer Journeys: Survivors Share Their Stories to Help Others.* Lincoln, NE: iUniverse, 2004.

Panno, Joseph, Ph.D. *Cancer: The Role of Genes, Lifestyle, and Environment.* New York, NY: Facts on File, 2004.

Sheen, Barbara. *Ovarian Cancer.* San Diego, CA: Lucent Books, 2005.

Teter, Becky, ed. *Torch: Tales of Remarkable Courage and Hope.* Dallas, TX: Baylor University, 2007.

Wyborny, Sheila. *Cancer Treatments.* Chicago, IL: Blackbirch, 2005.

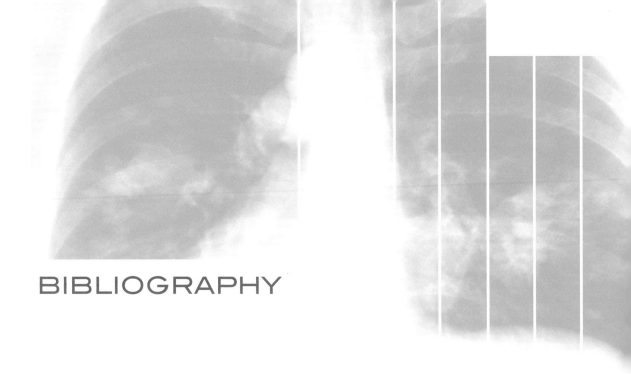

BIBLIOGRAPHY

American Cancer Society. "Cancer Facts and Figures 2007." Retrieved February 15, 2008 (http://www.cancer.org/downloads/STT/CAFF2007PWSecured.pdf).

Bourzac, Katherine. "Gene Therapy Without Viruses." *Technology Review*, Massachusetts Institute of Technology, September 12, 2007. Retrieved March 11, 2008 (http://www.technologyreview.com/Biotech/19367).

Cancer Research UK. "Chemotherapy for Ovarian Cancer." Retrieved March 2, 2008 (http://www.cancerhelp.org.uk/help/default.asp?page=3086).

Mayo Clinic. "Ovarian Cancer." Retrieved February 18, 2008 (http://www.mayoclinic.com/health/ovarian-cancer/DS00293).

Medline Plus. "Ovarian Cancer." Retrieved February 18, 2008 (http://www.nlm.nih.gov/medlineplus/ovariancancer.html#cat57).

Montz, F. J., and Robert E. Bristow. *A Guide to Survivorship for Women with Ovarian Cancer*. Baltimore, MD: Johns Hopkins University Press, 2005.

National Cancer Institute. "Ovarian Cancer." Retrieved February 20, 2008 (http://www.cancer.gov/cancertopics/types/ovarian),

Ohio State University Medical Center. "Ovarian Cancer and Hereditary Nonpolyposis Colon Cancer (HNPCC)." Retrieved March 2, 2008 (http://medicalcenter.osu.edu/patientcare/healthcare_services/gynecological_health/ovarian_cancer_hereditary_colon_cancer).

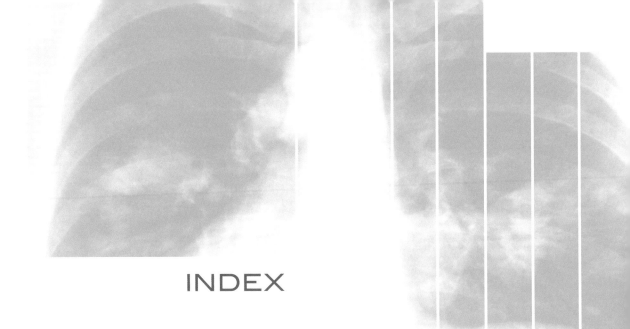

INDEX

ABOUT THE AUTHOR

Jeri Freedman earned a B.A. degree from Harvard University. For fifteen years, she worked for companies in the medical field. Among the numerous books she has written for young adults are *The Human Population and the Nitrogen Cycle*, *Hemophilia*, *Hepatitis B*, *Lymphoma: Current and Emerging Trends in Detection and Treatment*, *How Do We Know About Genetics and Heredity?*, *The Mental and Physical Effects of Obesity*, *Autism*, *Tay-Sachs Disease*, and *Applications and Limitations of Taxonomy in Classification of Organisms: An Anthology of Current Thought*.

PHOTO CREDITS

Designer: Evelyn Horovicz; Editor: Christopher Roberts;
Photo Researcher: Marty Levick